Research policies
for
health for all

World Health Organization
Regional Office for Europe
Copenhagen

Research policies
for
health for all

European Health for All Series, No. 2

ICP/RPD 110
Text editing by: M.S. Burgher

ISBN 92 890 1053 3

© World Health Organization 1988

PRINTED IN ENGLAND

CONTENTS

Preface

This book is the second in the new European Health for All Series. Like its predecessor,[a] its projected successors[b] and other publications from the Regional Office for Europe, it is aimed to help Member States in their work towards health for all by offering an up-to-the-minute response to current realities in the Region. Such a response is particularly important in the field of research, where technical and social developments have combined to make scientific investigation more complex, expensive and difficult — and its results more necessary and, potentially, more useful. The regional research strategy set out here, and the country strategies that Member States can tailor to their own needs and circumstances, can show countries how to improve health and shape a better future through a more effective investment of people, money and equipment in research.

The achievement of great social goals demands not only the political will to set the goals but also knowledge, as a basis for the action needed to reach them. In adopting the goal of health for all and the 38 regional targets as the means by which to reach it, the Member

---

[a] *Targets for health for all* (Copenhagen, WHO Regional Office for Europe, 1985 (European Health for All Series, No. 1)) contained the European health for all policy.

[b] These include the related publication *Priority research for health for all* (Copenhagen, WHO Regional Office for Europe, 1988 (European Health for All Series, No. 3)).

States of the WHO European Region have clearly demonstrated that they have the courage to pursue an ambitious vision. By endorsing target 32 — which requests countries to develop health research strategies to help realize this vision — the Member States have also acknowledged the value of research in producing the knowledge they need to take action.

In setting out a framework for a regional research strategy — a model for countries to adapt to their own use — this publication describes how, through research strategies, countries can use guided research on topics of high priority to generate and apply the information needed as the basis for action for health for all. Policymakers, at whom this publication is aimed, can promote research supportive of health for all development by establishing criteria for choosing research priorities and to ensure the provision of the prerequisites for successful investigations. This book suggests such criteria and details the prerequisites, along with ways of implementing a country policy and signs of its success. Although the publication speaks of country policies on research for health for all, it is understood that in most cases such a policy would be a component of a country's overall policy on health or on research.

The European Member States occupy a singularly good position for producing knowledge that can be used not only in the European Region but throughout the world to achieve health for all, owing to their vast research potential in universities, research institutions and WHO collaborating centres. There are obstacles, however, on the way. Many of these can be overcome through intersectoral collaboration. In particular, policies on research for health for all must be based on a new type of alliance between policy-makers and the research community. In this partnership each group will have new and complementary responsibilities, and both will gain, although society will benefit more. As policy-makers influence overall research priorities and use research findings to plan and run health care services and systems, they will make better use of a valuable tool to meet society's needs.

The research community in most countries, however, is independent and unaccustomed to gearing its activities, in part, to national policies. Nevertheless, promoting research for health for all, which some researchers may at first see as a threat, is actually an opportunity. Such research offers the chance to expand the domain of research to include fascinating virgin fields and methods of inquiry, along with new career opportunities, particularly for talented young investigators. In addition, research for health for all beckons the scientific community to a larger role in the political arena; researchers should participate in the making of the policy, influence the choice of priority areas for study and help to ensure that new information yielded by their research is put into practice more quickly and effectively through health care systems and services.

It is hoped that this publication will help Member States to continue their progress towards health for all by developing research strategies relevant to their own health policies and acceptable to their research communities. Such strategies require far better cooperation between policy-makers and the research community than currently exists in most countries. Together, both groups could work more effectively to provide knowledge and to use it for the achievement of the common goal: health for all. For this to happen it may be necessary to throw overboard some misconceptions that each party may have had about the other's role and effectiveness.

The time for action is now.

J.E. Asvall
*WHO Regional Director
for Europe*

Introduction

Knowledge is essential to transform a policy into a reality and research is the most powerful tool for generating this knowledge. Research — most often basic biomedical work on topics chosen by the investigators themselves — has supplied the knowledge behind the greatest victories in the fight against disease, disability and death. Such research is still undeniably valuable.

Nevertheless, the WHO Regional Office for Europe and the Member States of the Region are asking for a fundamental change in research. They ask that this tool be used more effectively than ever before, to reach a specific goal: health for all. They ask that policy-makers and the research community of each country work together to provide the knowledge needed to reach this goal, by building and using research strategies suited to their special needs.

Policy-makers and the research community in each Member State of the Region should cooperate to determine what research is most important, according to their own priorities, perform the studies and use the results to improve health. By taking up this challenge both groups will not just work more effectively; they will also make a better future for themselves and for society by helping to achieve health for all.

Health for all — global, regional and in countries — is the most ambitious health policy ever set. The Member States of WHO have chosen a far-reaching goal: health for all people by the year 2000.

Health for all through research

What health for all means

1

At the heart of the health for all movement is a new look at health with a broader perspective. Health remains the goal of health policies and health care systems, but it has a wider definition. The Member States have pledged to attain for their people more than a reduction in disease and disability. They are working for a positive kind of health: a state of complete physical, mental and social wellbeing. Reaching such a goal requires a wider view of the factors that affect health, encompassing something more than the physical problems of individual people. This view must examine the ways in which factors in society and in the environment affect people's health. A policy for health for all thus requires positive health to be built in new ways and new settings, by new combinations of people, in addition to the methods and means used successfully in the past.

The European Member States have taken the first steps towards their revolutionary goal. Through their representatives in the Regional Committee for Europe, the parliament of the Regional Office, they adopted 38 regional targets as concrete goals to work towards, and 65 regional indicators by which to measure their progress.[a] Briefly put, the targets describe how present conditions must be changed to reach health for all.

The 38 regional targets

The regional targets are not legal bonds on any Member State. They form a flexible framework that the political authorities, professional groups and general public of each nation can use to build their own targets, policies and programmes for health for all.

The targets have been carefully designed, and they fit as closely together as the blocks of stone that compose a pyramid. Each rests on the support of others and dovetails neatly with its neighbours. The apex of the pyramid is equity (target 1), to be attained by reducing present inequalities in health between and within countries.

The targets can be divided into three closely related groups, according to their purposes and their dates of completion. Fig. 1 illustrates this relationship.

---

[a] *Targets for health for all.* Copenhagen, WHO Regional Office for Europe, 1985 (European Health for All Series, No. 1).

2

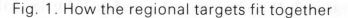
Fig. 1. How the regional targets fit together

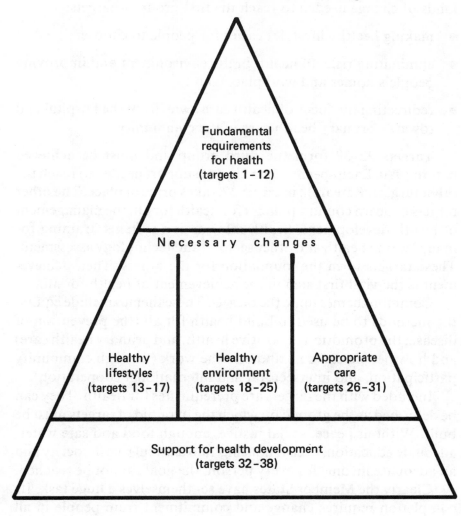

Fundamental
requirements
for health
(targets 1–12)

Necessary changes

Healthy
lifestyles
(targets 13–17)

Healthy
environment
(targets 18–25)

Appropriate
care
(targets 26–31)

Support for health development
(targets 32–38)

Targets 1–12 (to be achieved by the year 2000) are the fundamental requirements for health. These include equity, a longer and better life for all, and reductions in deaths from certain causes. Their achievement will mean that health for all is a reality.

3

Targets 13–31 (to be reached by 1995 or 1990) detail the three kinds of change needed to reach the first group of targets:

● making healthy lifestyles easier for people to choose;

● eliminating risks to health in the environment and improving people's homes and workplaces; and

● redirecting the focus of health care away from the hospital and towards primary health care in the community.

Targets 32–38 form the third group and must be achieved before 1990. Each specifies one kind of support needed to reach the other targets. Research, in target 32, takes pride of place. The other targets concern country policies for health for all, the management of health development, health information systems, training for manpower in health and other sectors, and technology assessment. These targets form the foundation for the others. Their achievement is the vital first step in the achievement of health for all.

Common themes unite the targets. These themes include equity, the methods to be used to build health for all (the prevention of disease, the promotion of positive health, and primary health care) and how people can contribute to the work (through community participation, and intersectoral and international cooperation).

Included with the targets are prerequisites for health. They can be described as the ground on which the pyramid of targets must be built. Without peace, social justice, enough food and safe water, adequate education, decent housing, and a useful role in society and an adequate income for every person, the goal cannot be reached.

Clearly the Member States have set themselves a huge task. Its completion requires change and commitment from people in all sectors of society in every Member State. People must discover how their work affects health and work actively with others for health for all. Five groups of people have rights to and responsibilities in health for all: health authorities at all levels (including policy-makers and administrators), health professionals of all kinds (including the research community), the people, sectors other than health, and international organizations.

4

This book discusses the responsibilities and opportunities for members of the first group in working through research for health for all. A related publication[a] sets out topics for such research.

The targets are to be achieved within a very short time (2–12 years). Action for health for all, based on knowledge, is plainly needed. Part of this knowledge already exists, and health for all would not be so far away if it were used. New knowledge is also needed. How to acquire and apply knowlege for health for all is a question that demands a response.

The Regional Committee's answer is target 32.

Before 1990, all Member States should have formulated research strategies to stimulate investigations which improve the application and expansion of knowledge needed to support their health for all developments.

This target can be achieved if Member States establish machinery to ensure the effective application of new knowledge in the development of health policies and programmes; determine what gaps there are in the knowledge needed to support the strategy of health for all and set research priorities accordingly; ensure a balanced representation of all academic disciplines relevant to health and of providers and users of health services as well as health policy-makers, in the planning and coordinating of research for health for all and make the research community an active contributor to the development of health for all; stimulate relevant multidisciplinary research; and allocate sufficient resources to conduct the research needed, giving preference to aspects that have not received the support they deserve.

In other words, the Member States of the Region have agreed that research strategies, resulting in guided research directed at

---

[a] *Priority research for health for all.* Copenhagen, WHO Regional Office for Europe, 1988 (European Health for All Series, No. 3).

specific goals, will ensure that the knowledge needed to attain health for all is provided and used well.

The targets cover fields of activity that are fundamental to public health but new subjects for country policies and health research. The structure of the targets suggests six broad tasks:

- describing every aspect of the health of the population so that progress towards the targets can be monitored (target 32);

- finding out what biological factors determine health (targets 1–12);

- assessing the part that lifestyles play in maintaining or endangering health (targets 13–17);

- studying the ways in which the physical, biological and social environment (including the basic prerequisites for health) determine the health of individuals and populations (targets 13–25);

- developing effective and efficient methods of providing people with appropriate care (targets 26–31); and

- improving policy-making, planning and management in programmes for health for all (targets 32–38).

To provide the necessary knowledge, health research must venture for the first time into fields that lie outside its traditional domain, the health and related sciences. To succeed, health researchers must seek cooperation with people in all the disciplines that can contribute the expert knowledge necessary. This will mainly involve the biomedical, behavioural and social sciences, although questions will also arise that will require answers from, for example, engineers, architects and other specialists.

Researchers working for health for all will take their expertise into new, unfamiliar areas and work with new colleagues in new ways. The research community has the chance not only to continue basic research for health but also, through goal-directed research, to take part directly in making and carrying out health and research policies. The research community can thus help to decide the future of its own profession by contributing to health for all.

When adopting the targets in 1984, the Regional Committee asked the European Advisory Committee on Health Research (EACHR) to help create a regional strategy for research for health for all. The EACHR (16 experts on different kinds of research, health administration, and research policies and administration) had two tasks: to advise the Regional Office for Europe on its regional policy on research for health for all, and to analyse each of the regional targets, to discover what kinds of research were most needed. In both tasks, the EACHR worked to meet three needs.

What research is needed?

The first was flexibility. Strategies for health for all must be carried out in all 32 Member States of the European Region, an area bounded by Norway in the north, Israel and Turkey in the south-east, the USSR in the east, Iceland in the north-west and Portugal in the south-west. All these countries have widely different patterns of mortality and morbidity, health care systems and research capacities. All must determine their own priorities and the regional research strategy must provide them with a framework and a guide for their own strategies.

The time frame for completing priority research had to be equally flexible. The completion dates set for the regional targets — some as early as 1990 — are far too restrictive to be applied to research. The regional strategy must point out areas of research that will contribute to achieving the targets, even if applicable results cannot be produced within such narrow time limits. A flexible time frame is particularly necessary to the opening of new areas of investigation.

Second, the regional strategy, and the analysis of the targets in particular, had to make specific recommendations for priority research to attain the targets. The EACHR therefore analysed the targets one by one, along with the Regional Committee's discussion of and suggestions for attaining them.

The third requirement was participation. Individual scientists, the scientific community, and national and international research bodies were all needed to take part in developing the regional strategy from the outset. They were to point out gaps in knowledge and the resulting needs for research. They were also to suggest, discuss and agree on both the research projects required and the timing of their implementation.

The work of the EACHR was considered by the Regional Committee, the Regional Health Development Advisory Council, the Consultative Group on Programme Development (15 senior health administrators who advise the WHO Regional Director for Europe on the regional programme), ministries of health, ministries responsible for science and technology, medical research councils, and by members of the research community, before it gained final approval from the Regional Committee at its thirty-seventh session in 1987. This book is one of the results.

Research strategies for Member States

Target 32 requests Member States to make research strategies to support their progress towards health for all. Like the regional targets, the regional research strategy presented here is an opportunity, not a prescription that all countries must follow to the letter. It should inspire European countries to develop research strategies that meet their priorities and needs by offering a framework on which they can construct their own research policies and projects. It is also designed to help countries to attain regional and country targets by translating them into concrete research recommendations, by enlisting the support of the research community for health for all, by guiding the allocation of research resources in Member States, and by stimulating all sectors to include health for all in their research policies. Finally, the regional strategy will guide the research activities of the Regional Office.

8

The regional strategy for research for health for all has three parts:

- an analysis of the most important research needs arising from the targets;

- a research policy that sets criteria for choosing research topics of high priority, and spells out the material and human resources needed and ways to ensure that they are provided; and

- a plan to promote and carry out the strategy.

Country strategies could have the same components.

This book discusses the implications of a research policy for the achievement of the targets, and a plan for promoting such a policy. The regional targets are analysed in detail, singly and in groups, for their research implications in the related publication, *Priority research for health for all*. Although specific research needs will vary from country to country, the targets themselves hint strongly at the kinds of research most useful in their achievement.

The work of the scientific community and health authorities, policy-makers and administrators cannot be separated for discussion as easily as the parts of a research strategy. While health authorities and the people who make health policy will be most concerned with this book and the scientific community is likely to be most interested in the companion publication, their roles are closely intertwined. As proof of the close relationship between both the subjects of and the audiences for the two books, the publications have an introduction and first chapter in common.

Just as community participation is a cornerstone of health for all, so cooperation between and within both groups is essential to the success of strategies for research for health for all. An effective strategy demands that policy-makers and researchers help each other to fulfil their complementary roles. Policy-makers should point out important topics for research. Researchers should not only study these, but advise policy-makers on their choices and help to make both research policy and plans for using the knowledge gained. Policy-makers should then use these findings to plan and run health care systems and services. Finally, researchers should evaluate the success of the whole strategy.

By working together within the regional and country research strategies, policy-makers and the research community can produce not only vital knowledge for health for all but also the kind of intersectoral collaboration that will help to make it a reality.

The regional analysis: a framework for setting priorities

This summary of the regional analysis of the targets for health for all identifies the areas of research needed to attain them. Just as health for all calls upon the scientific community to take part in research policy, so policy-makers can profit from the discussion of priority areas of research. While the regional analysis displays an inventory of tempting opportunities to the scientific community, it also carries implications for research policy by suggesting priorities among the different topics. These priorities will be particularly interesting to the people in charge of policy on health research at country level. The regional analysis is a starting point from which researchers and makers of country policies on research for health for all can take their first step: choosing their own priorities.

In analysing each of the 38 regional targets, the European Advisory Committee on Health Research worked to stimulate research of priority in the struggle to achieve regional and country targets, not all possible research related to health. The members of the Committee tried to choose research topics that are:

Choosing priority areas for research

- highly likely to contribute to the attainment of the regional targets (preferably but not exclusively within the time frame suggested by the Regional Committee);

- closely linked to the Regional Committee's suggested solutions for attainment,[a] although other options will be pursued;

- likely to yield results that can be translated into health policy and action; and

- unfortunately, likely to be neglected otherwise, despite their importance.

The Member States themselves pinpointed gaps in knowledge and problems in achieving the targets in the first of their triennial evaluations of their progress towards health for all.[b]

Common themes   The regional targets share common themes, vital elements of their success: equity, disease prevention, health promotion, primary health care, community participation, and intersectoral and international cooperation. Similar themes run through research for health for all. They include three areas of research:

— health policy and organizational behaviour

— inequities

— community participation and intersectoral collaboration

and two essential tools:

— better information systems and indicators for the targets

— international comparative studies.

Naturally, many concrete research questions can touch several themes. The importance of the themes will, of course, vary from country to country.

---

[a] Solutions for attaining the targets are thoroughly discussed in *Targets for health for all* (Copenhagen, WHO Regional Office for Europe, 1985 (European Health for all Series, No. 1)).

[b] *Evaluation of the strategy for health for all by the year 2000. Seventh report on the world health situation. Vol. 5: European Region.* Copenhagen, WHO Regional Office for Europe, 1986.

Research on health policy and organizational behaviour is an overriding priority for four main reasons.

First, although enough information is already available to take firm action on many targets, nothing is being done. Research on implementation is therefore needed. Most of the problems of, obstacles to and constraints on implementation can be understood by applying the concepts and methods of such disciplines as political science, sociology, social policy and management science. In addition, policy formulation should be systematically scrutinized as a social process. This is a difficult area of study. In implementation analysis, in particular, the researcher must deal with vested interests and the inevitable problems arising from the definitions used. Researchers must also have the courage not only to recognize that no further information is needed but to tell policy-makers that the time has come for action.

Second, current health care systems do not function as well as they should. In many important areas, current services are based on conventional wisdom rather than hard scientific evidence. Health systems research and evaluative research can help to show the best way to deliver services. Technology assessment will allow people to choose technology (equipment, drugs and procedures) of proven safety, efficiency, effectiveness and acceptability. Finally, quality assurance will see that high standards of care are met.

Third, the regional targets detail changes in the organization of health care systems and emphasize community participation in and consumer satisfaction with health services as keys to health for all. The targets call for several far-reaching structural changes. These include: a shift of emphasis from the hospital to primary health care as the focus of health care, more teamwork among health personnel, more systematic mechanisms for quality assurance and technology assessment, the promotion of more effective community participation, the encouragement of mutual-aid groups, and the introduction of systematic planning for research. Such changes must be founded on knowledge of the conditions, constraints and consequences of organizational development.

13

Fourth, the direction of health research needs to be scrutinized. Researchers are usually more interested in providing better means to reach the goals of social and health policies than in questioning these goals. Now may be the time to make a critical analysis of the goals of research, particularly research on health systems. Such work often focuses more on the quality, accessibility and cost-efficiency of services and systems than on their effects on health, acceptability, and ethical and political desirability.

Priority research on health policy and organizational behaviour should address:

- the relationship between overall social policy goals, health policy and people's health;

- influences on the design and implementation of health policy;

- the means of carrying out health policy and the priority ranking of health policy goals;

- the role of other sectors in health care;

- the relationship between official and unofficial (professional and lay) care systems and between public and private care sectors;

- the organizational and administrative structures of central, regional and local health care;

- the cost–benefit ratio, cost-efficiency and cost-effectiveness of new and established health services; and

- the quality of care.

Inequities　　Target 1 deals with equity in health. This is no accident; raising the overall level of health and increasing equity are the two basic goals of health care. People may suffer from inequities because of their social status or class, sex, ethnic group or geographic location. Despite the position of equity as the pinnacle of the targets, establishing a reliable picture of equity within and between countries will be very difficult until they improve their information base on this critical issue.

14

Research on equity should include:

- defining concepts and creating indicators to measure inequities in health;

- gaining a better understanding of the factors and mechanisms that create and maintain inequities; and

- studying policies and evaluating programmes to reduce health inequities.

Community participation and intersectoral collaboration, themes of the regional targets, are two of the cornerstones of all work for health for all. Relatively little is known, however, about how they have been organized. Less is known about their effects on the cost, effectiveness, quality and acceptability of health policies and services. Even the idea of community participation is poorly defined. Studies on such questions are urgently needed. Determining the role of community participation in primary health care is particularly important.

Community participation and intersectoral collaboration

Better information is so urgently needed that one of the targets is devoted to it. Today's information systems do not provide the kinds of information necessary to achieve the targets or to measure progress towards achieving them. Weaknesses can be found in: the definition of concepts of and boundaries between sectors of health care, and the availability, reliability and interpretation of data. It is also difficult to disaggregate data in a way that makes them relevant to various population, administrative and geographical groups. Finally, the length, techniques and coverage of reporting vary among countries.

Need for better information

Current data also say very little about such problems in health care as the quality of life, overtreatment, iatrogenic disease, the feelings of alienation in patients and their families, the unwanted extension of life, or the emotional and financial costs of illness to the family. Further, present information systems are not well suited to assessing equity.

15

This problem calls for two remedies: the development of better information systems, and, within these, the development of better indicators for evaluating progress.

Research is needed to standardize procedures for data collection and to assess the cost-effectiveness of collecting new data. A balance must also be struck between the legitimate needs of policy-makers and researchers for information and the protection of patients' rights to privacy and confidentiality.

Health information systems. Most health information systems have been designed to collect administrative data. They are often simple "head counts" showing, for example, how much money has been spent or how many surgical operations have been performed.

The usefulness of the information collected can be increased in two ways. First, the value of a single item of data can be enhanced by making it more detailed and precise or by adding modifiers to derive secondary data. For example, the severity of conditions could be recorded along with diagnoses or a price tag or estimate could be attached to the record of each service used. Cost-analysis or time-and-motion studies may be needed to obtain such modifiers. Second, several items of data can be combined in various ways to provide more meaningful information.

Looking at the relationships between data will produce useful information for health planning, evaluation and health service research. More must be known than the total number of services produced; research must reveal the impact of care on people's health — not just the number of patients discharged but their satisfaction with their care. Other neglected areas are the safety and acceptability of procedures to patients and the cost-effectiveness of services. Information systems should also allow researchers to identify and analyse differences in health care practices.

Indicators. Developing a standard system of collecting information is one of the most pressing needs in research for health for all. This system should be applied to all the kinds of data that are relevant to achieving the targets but either unavailable at present or

16

interpreted differently from country to country. Research must focus on the types of data that should be collected; how to define, store, retrieve and evaluate them; and what kinds of feedback mechanism must be established to monitor specific programmes.

New indicators of health need to be developed or existing ones must be improved in several areas.[a] Equity is perhaps the most important, but problems that cross national boundaries also deserve special attention. Most indicators on these issues are qualitative; quantitative indicators should complement them whenever possible. The possibilities for disaggregating data in a meaningful way should be increased. The variables used in the disaggregation should have clear, standard definitions.

New or better indicators are also needed to assess:

- the consumer's view of health care needs;
- early changes in biological systems caused by long-term, low-dose exposure to environmental agents;
- the effectiveness of health care services (results, quality of care, client satisfaction);
- the costs and efficiency of services;
- community participation in health care;
- health behaviour and positive health; and
- the evaluation of health systems development (through the use of "tracers").

The targets call for many profound changes. Such reforms can be risky and costly ventures. The political risks may be great because the outcome cannot always be guaranteed. Policy-makers may

International comparative studies

---

[a] A revision of the regional indicators has been endorsed by the Regional Committee for Europe: *Revised list of indicators and procedure for monitoring progress towards health for all in the European Region (1987–1988)* (Copenhagen, WHO Regional Office for Europe, 1987 (unpublished document EUR/RC37/8 Rev.1)).

want to know about the experience of other countries, particularly if the countries are engaged in similar activities. Such information is often difficult to obtain. It may not be be collected systematically; many variables of interest to other countries may be overlooked. Finally, the information may be unavailable simply because of language barriers or because it is scattered throughout the system.

International comparative studies can help to solve these problems. They can give better insights into many aspects of progress towards health for all than studies conducted within a single country. They are particularly useful in working for appropriate care. Traditions in care and the organization of health services can often be better evaluated when contrasted with those of other countries, where their development has taken a different direction.

Much can be learned from an analysis of the strengths and weaknesses of different countries' approaches to organizing health care. Studies based on rigorous scientific research designs, however, not only are very expensive but also yield results that may be difficult to use. Fortunately, relatively simple and inexpensive descriptive studies may be wholly sufficient for decision-making.

Regular international health surveys might be another solution to the problems of method and expense. The surveys could be carried out in connection with or as a complement to the triennial regional evaluations of progress towards health for all, to avoid duplication of work. To minimize costs and lighten the burden on countries of collecting data, health surveys could cover a sample of Member States and their populations. Although each survey should include certain basic measurements, to enable trends to be assessed, it should also have its own specific focus. Each country should use similar definitions and standardized measurements, to produce comparable results.

International collaborative studies are needed:

● to collate, compare and disseminate the information available in different countries on the strengths and weaknesses of various approaches to providing health services and on many other variables related to the regional targets;

- to carry out truly comparative research according to a common protocol, to study most of the areas related to achieving the regional targets, particularly the area of health policy; and

- to provide models for developing health services.

At the beginning of this book, the 38 regional targets were compared to a pyramid (Fig. 1) because the attainment of each will result from or lead to the attainment of others. Further, the structure they form will lead to a peak of achievement: equity in health. Like architects explaining a design, people explaining the targets begin at the top. They start by discussing the great goal and the other targets that form the 12 fundamental requirements for health for all in Europe. Then they talk about how to get there: through the three groups of necessary changes (healthy lifestyles, a healthy environment and appropriate care). They finish by examining the foundation of the structure, the seven kinds of support needed to make the necessary changes.

This is the right way to describe a plan or a completed project. The European Member States, however, are moving from the first to the second position. They have begun the work to achieve the targets, but it is far from over. To build this monument, the countries of Europe are working from the ground up.

For this reason, the regional analysis of the targets begins with the foundation for health for all, the last group of targets, which are to be attained first. This group starts, appropriately enough, with research. The discussion then moves through appropriate care, a healthy environment and healthy lifestyles and ends with the fundamental requirements for health.

This order has some interesting features. For example, research grows in importance as the reader moves from group to group. In addition, the reader parallels the journey that researchers and policy-makers will take as they expand their familiar responsibilities to include the new opportunities in health for all.

Some of the landmarks on this journey are familiar. For example, the bulk of health research is already proceeding, most

19

often successfully, towards many of the same goals as the first 12 targets. Why, then, should the Member States and the research community take on the arduous job of working through the targets? The answer lies in the nature of the health for all movement. It is designed not to reject but to build on the successes of the past and present, to reach a more complete kind of health in the future. This means that research will be sharpened and refined and therefore a more effective tool in the work for positive health.

Although research priorities will vary from one country to another, on the basis of the target-by-target analysis, the following summary of overall priorities for each of the five groups of targets may be suggested for Europe as a whole.

Support for health development (targets 32–38)

The last seven targets detail a number of prerequisites for all work to improve health, including research. These requirements must be met to change attitudes and working practices among politicians, health authorities, health personnel, people in other sectors and, above all, the general public. One prerequisite — research strategies (target 32) — is so important that it is the subject of this book. Another — the need for more detailed, reliable and standardized data for every target (target 34) — is an overriding theme of research for health for all. The other necessary kinds of support are: country health policies committed to the principles of health for all, well trained and motivated health personnel, support from professions outside the health sector, and health care technology that meets people's needs in an effective and an acceptable way.

Increased research is needed for:

— making health policy

— educating health personnel

— assessing health technology.

Health policies based on the principles of health for all can probably best be promoted by a clear demonstration of their advantages: greater effectiveness, efficiency and equity. Therefore, comparative studies, policy research, scenarios and simulation

20

models are needed to determine which health care systems can best meet the goal of improving people's health at minimal cost and in an equitable way.

Ironically, the success of modern health care has created the need to change the education of health personnel. Acute conditions are losing ground to chronic and disabling health problems. The aging of the population will reinforce this trend. The central question here is how to adapt the education of health personnel to the new health needs of the chronically ill, the elderly, the mentally ill and long-term patients. Cultural and recreational needs should be included with needs for medical care. Evaluative research on existing training programmes should compare their objectives (and results) with the new objectives, skills and attitudes required to meet actual health care needs. Different models of education for health personnel should be compared, to point out the curricula and teaching methods most likely to improve health workers' abilities and motivation to provide competent, comprehensive care in the community.

The tendency towards an unchecked expansion of health technology brings a number of evils in its train. The costs of care skyrocket, the providers and users of services are alienated from one another, and patients are treated like objects and lose their responsibility for their own health. The assessment of health technology can control the tendency and fight its unfortunate side effects. Multidisciplinary research is urgently needed at all levels to improve the assessment of health technology.

The work should begin with deciding what technology most needs assessment and setting criteria to make such decisions. Next, the technology selected must be evaluated for its efficacy, efficiency and impact on society. Finally, the study results must be built into coherent recommendations for health policy, and these recommendations must be used to change the practice of health care and health care planning.

These six targets outline the design and structure of a system for the delivery of appropriate health care, based on well developed,

Appropriate care (targets 26–31)

21

integrated primary health care. The quality of care should be assured through the systematic assessment of technology and evaluations of health workers' performance. Appropriate care is so important in achieving health for all that it is a basic theme of the targets and a priority in research that has already been discussed in part.

Successfully redirecting a health care system primarily depends on political will and decision-making. Research on health systems can be an important source of advice for policy-makers. It can also help to ease the transition from the hospital to primary health care as the centre of health care systems. Researchers can draw policy-makers' attention to considerable amounts of existing data.

The central research questions are:

- how to develop a system of primary health care adapted to countries' central and local circumstances;

- how to allocate resources according to people's needs;

- how to achieve a proper balance of resources between primary health care and hospital and specialized care;

- how to mobilize community participation;

- how to educate health care personnel in teamwork and the management of services;

- how to make primary health care more acceptable to patients and how to use it to support lay care and self-help; and

- how to assess the quality of care and how to use the results to improve the acceptability of health services to patients and the feedback to health personnel.

Healthy environment (targets 18–25)
These eight targets have two aims, as closely related as the two sides of a coin. The first is to safeguard human health from potential harm resulting from biological, chemical and physical agents, including hazardous waste. The second is to enhance the quality of life by providing people with clean water and air, safe food, and pleasant living and working conditions.

22

Increased research is needed to:

— study specific agents and their effects

— provide information on risks and their management

— develop integrated monitoring systems

— promote community participation in work for environmental health.

More basic research is needed on health hazards in the environment, their causes and possible means of preventing them. This work should include studies on genetic variability, ecogenetics and environmental genotoxicology. The interaction of different agents has to be investigated at the level of the intact animal, the organ and the cellular and subcellular systems. Other important topics are the interaction of low-dose and long-term exposure to agents and combined exposure to various risks.

A comprehensive and internationally comparable inventory is needed of the available data on both environmental agents and their effects on the environment and health. Such an inventory should also review the data for their usefulness in preventing environmental risks and protecting health. The data collected should include facts that will help political decision-makers to manage risks and to improve regulations and laws to protect the environment.

Sometimes the best way of protecting human health may be to monitor the environment. At other times, it may be better to monitor adverse effects in the population, preferably before symptoms are recognized. Monitoring must cover all aspects of environmental health in which risk management is called for. Research must show what is to be monitored and how this should be done to ensure that the information is valuable in decision-making.

Finally, the public must be encouraged to take a greater part in presenting, discussing and handling environmental health issues. Studies based on the behavioural and social sciences must identify ways to provide people with better information on health concerns and risk factors. They must also show how to establish community

23

participation in environmental risk management. This will result in a greater desire for safety, and decision-makers will take greater care to ensure that they consider environmental health when planning and assessing new developments.

Lifestyles conducive to health (targets 13–17)

Lifestyles (which are largely determined by the individual, societal and environmental factors that prevail in a society and the different groups composing it) strongly influence health or illness. The five targets on lifestyles recognized these facts. The social and behavioural sciences have two important roles in research on lifestyles. They should assess the effects of various lifestyles on health and promote the concept of healthy lifestyles as the normal way of life in a society.

Increased research is needed on:

— indicators of lifestyles

— lifestyles that damage health (risk behaviour)

— lifestyles that improve health (positive health behaviour)

— induced changes in lifestyle (health promotion).

Valid, reliable and sensitive indicators of health-related behaviour are needed to discover exactly how lifestyles affect health. In particular, completely new measures should be developed to assess such factors as positive health behaviour, social support and social integration, and chronic stress arising from work and from roles imposed on people according to their sex.

Intervention programmes must be based on a thorough understanding of what health-damaging behaviour does to the person who engages in it, and the purpose it serves for the individual and society. Research can provide the knowledge needed. In addition, all intervention programmes should be scientifically evaluated.

The emphasis on positive health is a promising new approach to improving people's health. It implies a fundamental change of direction for health research: a shift from the study of disease and treatment to the study of health and factors that promote it. A clearer concept of positive health is urgently needed. Descriptive

24

and analytical studies of how certain lifestyles can benefit health are equally important.

The deepest motive for studying current lifestyles is the intention to change them, to promote lifestyles that enhance health and to reduce those that damage it. Large-scale attempts to modify widespread behaviour will, however, cause ethical and practical problems. These can be solved only if new forms of community participation are developed for planning and running intervention programmes and the research projects that will accompany them.

Targets 1–12 aim at reducing health inequities, morbidity and mortality from specific causes, and at improving the quality of life.

Fundamental requirements for health for all (targets 1–12)

Increased research is needed:

— to improve the data base

— to redirect research towards public health needs

— in the forms of longitudinal studies and small area data.

Setting up a reliable data base on inequities, morbidity, mortality and the quality of life is of primary importance. It is needed to provide information for the monitoring of progress towards the targets.

Priority should be given to research projects aimed at prevention of, treatment of or rehabilitation for common diseases. Research that offers chances of improving the quality of life is equally important. Research objectives should not therefore be limited to issues affecting only selected target populations, such as hospital patients, but should extend to problems of morbidity in primary care and the community. While better, broader assessments of high-powered modern technology are urgently needed, more attention should also be paid to diagnostic and therapeutic strategies and evaluative research in primary health care.

Chronic, disabling disease causes many major public health problems in the European Region, which will be augmented by the aging of the population. Research is urgently needed on the course and outcome of different forms of illness over periods of years, the relevant risk factors, and the effectiveness of different forms of intervention, even though the results of such studies may not be available by the target date.

To give a wider focus to health policy, health surveys should include people's perceptions of their health and that of their families. Both retrospective and, in most cases, prospective longitudinal studies will also be necessary. Small area data on the need for health services, and their provision and results, are required to plan and evaluate intervention programmes. These data should be collated with relevant community or regional data.

2

Research policies

Countries need policies on research for health for all. Everyone affected by such a policy — researchers, science and research authorities, health authorities, and people in other relevant sectors and in the community — should take part in creating it. It should function as an integral part of two other policies: a country policy on health research and a country policy on health for all. At the start, these will be two different things.

First, a country's policy on general health research is concerned with all health research, not with the specific needs for knowledge for health for all. Second, Member States are responding to target 33, which urges them to bring their health policies and strategies into line with the principles of health for all, by creating their own policies for health for all. As countries progress towards the goal, of course, these two kinds of policy will draw closer together. A policy on research for health for all can do vital service for both.

The value of such a policy to the success of an overall policy for health for all is obvious, but it could give equally valuable support to general policies on health research. Relatively few countries have them; research policies for health for all could be the seeds from which general health research policies could grow.

Four developments in society and in research make a general policy on health research very attractive. General policies on health research can help solve the problems posed by these changes or even

The need for general health research policies

27

turn them to advantage. These changes demand that research change, too. The focus must shift, in part, from work generated by the researcher to guided research designed to meet society's needs. Changing the direction of research will, however, take a long time. As a Chinese proverb says, if a tree takes a thousand years to grow, one must not waste a day in planting it. Research policies are needed now, if they are to direct the future of research.

Rapid change is a fact of life in today's society. A general health research policy could help ensure that social change results from planning and adaptation, not from a series of crises. Scientific research could provide the basis for action to change society, and monitoring and control could help planners anticipate or avoid the negative consequences of such changes. Through a general health research policy, planners could help direct social change, not merely respond to it.

Scarce resources are another fact of life. A research policy could help to see that the research community receives its share of available resources and uses them wisely, by devoting them to research studies whose results would support major social policies such as health for all.

Further, more and more people want a voice in making decisions that affect them. WHO has acknowledged both the demand for community participation and its potential usefulness by making the people's participation a cornerstone of the work for health for all. A research policy can satisfy this demand and make research more effective by giving the people who will use the results (or be affected by them) the chance to help decide research priorities and, if possible, to help design and conduct the studies.

Finally, research is growing in many senses. The broader understanding of health and the factors that influence it has resulted in multidisciplinary and interdisciplinary projects that often employ increasing numbers of researchers. Because much equipment has a shorter average working life, it must be replaced more often and at greater cost. Improved information systems produce more data on more phenomena than ever before. Computers and refined methods of analysis allow these data to be analysed in versatile ways. In

28

addition, some types of research, such as genetic engineering, may have unintended and undesirable consequences.

A general research policy can help society deal with (and even profit from) the increasing scale, complexity, expense and potential usefulness of current research. Through such a policy, potential problems could be anticipated. Perhaps they could be avoided or even become opportunities. Changes in research have made it a more powerful but more unwieldy tool. A general policy on health research — in other words, thinking harder about the goals of research — can allow a country to control and use this tool more effectively for the good of society.

Similarly, a research policy for health for all would mean that policy-makers were thinking harder about how to use research to pave the way to health for all.

All the regional targets will not be equally important in all countries. Member States will usually choose their own priorities from the targets and set targets of their own. A country's policy on research for health for all should therefore aim at systematically analysing the targets given highest priority in that country to determine how research can help to achieve them (Fig. 2). The regional analysis of the targets provides a framework and starting point for such analysis in Member States. The analysis of a target may reveal:

Why a country policy on research for health for all?

- that research is not needed; or

- that research is needed, either to help apply available knowledge or to generate new knowledge.

The first question to be asked in such an analysis is whether the target has already been reached. If the answer is yes, it may be useful to determine how this was done and set a new, more ambitious target. If the answer is no, the next question is: Can knowledge help to close the gap between the target and reality? Even if the answer is no, it may be necessary to find the reasons for this gap. They could include prevailing social values, lack of

29

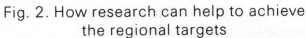

Fig. 2. How research can help to achieve the regional targets

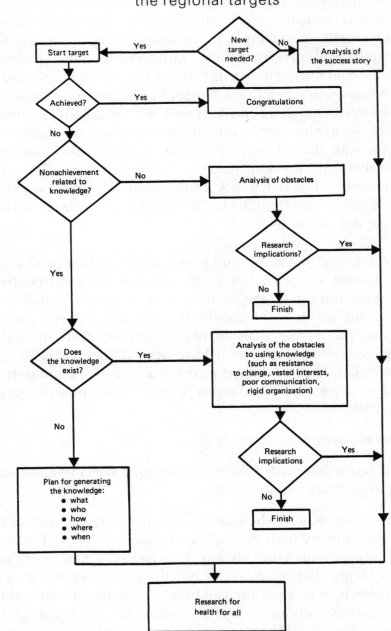

resources, poor organization, lack of motivation, insufficient collaboration between different sectors or resistance from vested interests. Research can solve many of these problems.

If problems related to knowledge seem to be the cause of the gap, the next question is: Does the knowledge exist? A positive answer should lead to a scrutiny of the reasons why it is not being used.

A negative answer brings us to the core of a country policy on research for health for all. What is the best, most cost-effective way to achieve the targets through knowledge? This question raises a whole series of new ones, which a successful country policy must answer.

- Exactly what knowledge is needed to reach the targets?

- Who would be best suited to carry out this research?

- Do researchers need further training?

- Are the organization and settings for research optimal?

- Are the resources (money, people and equipment) available?

- Do appropriate methods exist?

- What should be done to ensure that new knowledge is used in decision-making and programme implementation?

Although policies on research for health for all will differ from country to country, all successful policies will share several features.

Features of a country policy

People from a wide range of disciplines must be involved in the development and implementation of a country policy on research for health for all. Involving researchers in policy development from the very beginning will circumvent many obstacles and misunderstandings that might otherwise develop between policy-makers and researchers. While such a policy can, at first, be developed on its own, it must ultimately be fully incorporated in both the country's general health research policy and its policy for health for all.

31

A policy on research for health for all needs to be practical and scientifically sound. It must be written in clear, nonbureaucratic language understood by the research community. Otherwise, both health for all and the research related to it may look like impractical dreams.

Finally, a country policy must have a strong evaluation component, to guide its further development by systematically appraising its results. As countries move at different speeds towards the achievement of health for all, their priorities and research needs will change. A country policy on research for health for all has to be open to feedback on both research and implementation. All those concerned — the health and research authorities and the research community — must periodically evaluate the policy and revise it accordingly. Researchers must be assured that the policy is a versatile tool, not a straitjacket.

Tasks for policy-makers

Member States naturally have different overall needs in health research and specific needs to achieve regional and country targets. Nevertheless, policy-makers in all countries should use policies on research for health for all to achieve two goals: the setting of priorities for future research and the establishment of ways to guarantee the prerequisites for successful research.

Setting priorities for research

Setting priorities means taking three steps:

● specifying the criteria for setting research priorities and obtaining consensus on their use;

● identifying neglected areas of research (including economic, ethical and philosophical issues) that should receive higher priority; and

● establishing goals and setting priorities.

The first step is the most important, as it will determine the direction of the other two.

The following could be useful criteria. Priority research for health for all should be:

- carried out on problems with high human, social and economic cost and of epidemiological significance (in avoidable mortality, morbidity or disability);

- relevant to the achievement of the regional or country targets;

- scientifically sound and significant;

- likely to be successfully performed;

- likely to improve health care practice; and

- likely to be cost-effective or to guarantee that resources already invested will yield results.

Of course, other considerations in setting research priorities include: the organization of the health care system, available health resources, genetic factors, social values, cultural norms and other factors in each country.

The second task of a country policy on research for health for all — providing resources for priority research and ensuring the use of the findings — requires:

Prerequisites for priority research

- determining the needs for education and training of personnel that emerge from the suggested priorities;

- guaranteeing the material prerequisites and manpower for research;

- establishing a funding policy;

- allocating resources according to the goals and priorities; and

- making research findings easy for planners, decision-makers and other researchers to use.

The most important prerequisites for priority research can be divided into groups: incentives, financing, personnel development, organization and communication. Incentives will attract talented researchers. Adequate financing, personnel development and changes in the organization of research will allow researchers to do the work needed. They are, therefore, also incentives to research for health for all. The final prerequisite is communication. It is essential not only among researchers but also between researchers and the people who will use their findings.

Incentives. The research community cannot be expected to take research for health for all seriously unless the highest authorities in each country demonstrate their commitment to health for all and to a research policy through statements showing a clear political will. In federal countries, such commitment may be needed at regional or other levels. Bodies responsible for running or making policy on research, such as central research councils, could make corresponding statements. Such statements could help give prestige to the kinds of research needed to achieve the targets, and attract researchers to the work.

In addition, scientists from different disciplines are much more likely to perform priority research for health for all if they have a say in setting priorities and designing the research. Scientific groups and professional associations should help to develop and update country strategies for research for health for all. They should also review research protocols. As a result, they will become more interested in the work and encourage young investigators to take part. The involvement of the scientific community will lead to a greater number of articles on research for health for all, and these will be more acceptable to scientific journals. In turn, the publishing of the findings of such research will give it more prestige.

Research has traditionally been conducted in universities. Although expressions of political commitment will help to secure their support, other incentives will increase their chances of making a useful contribution. These will include the provision of necessary resources and, possibly, administrative changes that will help people in different disciplines to work together. Special research institutes, new professorships and postgraduate training pro- grammes, particularly research training programmes, have often helped to promote new fields. Academic researchers should, when possible, also have service attachments. If they give health care or work in a hospital or primary health care centre, they can avoid succumbing to "the ivory tower syndrome" that can make their work useless to others.

A change of attitude and structure within the health care system is another necessary incentive. Although much research for health for all needs to be carried out as an integral part of the normal work of the health care system, many administrators and employers within the system — as well as some researchers — think it has no place there. Perhaps the most effective way of changing their attitude is to show, through success stories, that research can indeed produce results that are useful both in political decision- making and in planning and running health services. Action must follow this change. Structures are needed to enable research to be done within the health care system and to promote cooperation between researchers and the people in charge of health and social welfare services.

Finally, talented researchers should be able to make careers in working for health for all. This requirement is often particularly difficult to meet for social scientists. In addition, administrative changes should allow both care providers and academics (particu- larly clinicians and clinical teachers) to make research a part of their usual duties. Possibilities should be explored for ensuring sufficient time and adequate working conditions for such part-time researchers.

Financing. Adequate resources, both money and equipment, are one of the best incentives to research in any field; they should be allocated according to the country policy on research for health for all. A lack of sufficient funding could set up a vicious circle: limited research and development result in low status, rewards and morale; high-quality staff cannot be recruited; good research cannot be done; and status and morale sink lower. Increased funding is thus needed for research for health for all. It should come from new sources; reallocating funds currently given to health research should be only a last resort.

Social security, private foundations and industry need to join government in contributing funds, as they, too, will profit from the success of health for all. Attracting the interest of private foundations, particularly to research on topics not covered by direct or indirect government funding, is essential. Better coordination is needed between funding agencies (which could form a joint advisory council) and between the ministries concerned (which could meet periodically to discuss research policy). Possibilities for raising funds from lower levels of government could also be considered.

Personnel development. The greatest bottleneck in carrying out the research needed is a lack of trained people, not of money. Research reports often show that studies are not based on fully satisfactory research designs or do not employ the most up-to-date methods. Training in community and social medicine, epidemiology, statistics, computer science and research methods offers a partial remedy to the problem. Other specific areas in which training should be stepped up are social sciences related to health, systems analysis, operational research, geriatrics, toxicology, environmental risk assessment and health economics. To be able to run multidisciplinary projects, researchers also need training in management.

Further, research workers should have the chance to take advantage of available research training. They could, for example, be granted at least partly paid leaves of absence or sabbaticals.

In many areas, the demand for research training is too small to justify a programme within one country. International collaboration on training (among WHO, research councils, academies of science, foundations and other similar bodies) could be the answer.

Organization. Research to attain the targets should be incorporated into existing research programmes and use available expert knowledge. Research centres or groups with experience in the relevant fields should be encouraged to cooperate and contribute to the development of research capabilities in countries.

New forms of cooperation between the sciences are needed to establish fertile ground for the multidisciplinary work essential to research for health for all. Such research can only flourish where there is easy access to different kinds of expertise and when all participants are considered equal. Some of the organizational walls separating different disciplines (and hindering communication and cooperation) must be levelled.

Universities could provide a particularly favourable environment. They are reservoirs of talent and intellectual and technical competence in many fields. They could:

- develop programmes to train personnel in new forms of research and in applying research findings in health care services;

- help individuals, other universities and related institutions, organizations and countries to exchange information, experience, and research plans, programmes and findings;

- standardize the methods of interdisciplinary research as well as the indicators used to determine health status and define health problems; and

- set up research working groups to cut across the boundaries between disciplines and professions and to determine and attack obstacles to success.

Because universities can secure cooperation among scientific institutions, a European network of universities, established by WHO, could give immeasurable aid in the tasks whose completion demands international cooperation. Such a network may have a particularly important part in achieving the regional targets. Health services research centres could also contribute.

Science administrations should be organized in a way that allows them to respond to society's basic health needs and to support its policies, such as those for health for all. For instance, all relevant disciplines must be represented in a country's medical research council. Such councils may have to be established on a regional level in federal countries. In many countries, health and science and research are the responsibilities of different ministries. As a result, the links between the health authorities and those responsible for research and science are too weak for effective cooperation. Changing this division of labour may be unnecessary or impossible, but communication between authorities could certainly be improved.

Communication. The importance of communication in carrying out research for health for all has already been mentioned. It is perhaps even more necessary in ensuring that the results of the work reach the people who need them.

The results of research for health for all are intended for immediate use in planning and running health care systems and services. In many countries, the links between research and health policy are not strong enough. On the one hand, policy-makers and health professionals do not systematically review and use either the existing or the new knowledge generated by research. On the other, many researchers are ignorant of key issues and developments in health policy. Research workers seldom point out the practical implications of their work, and decision-makers and even health professionals seldom use scientific knowledge to support their decisions.

Communication between researchers and health policy-makers and professionals is vital. Each should have a better understanding of the others' needs. Opportunities for each to see the others at work, as well as special events intended to bring the groups together to discuss ways of applying current research, would help improve communication.

Researchers and decision-makers and administrators should make special efforts to identify and remove the obstacles to communication between them. In fact, each group should try to reach out to the others. Users of research results should search for them and the research community should recognize the need to spread the news of their work not only in scientific journals but also in publications read by decision-makers and administrators. Research findings must be presented in language comprehensible to all who will use them. New journals may be needed to cater to the common needs of researchers, decision-makers and administrators. Further, projects for research relevant to policy-making should include a publishing plan to meet the needs of the different people who will use the knowledge to be generated.

WHO has always turned to research for advice and answers. What part can the scientific community take in policies on research for health for all? The members of the scientific community have three major responsibilities in generating new knowledge.

Work for the scientific community

First, research workers must share the results of their work with decision-makers, for use in revising health care practices. They must also help spread new knowledge by presenting it to others in the scientific community for critical and constructive discussion. This will safeguard decision-makers against misleading information, dishonesty or unbalanced judgements. Researchers must also present their findings to the public in a clear and useful form. In addition, they and other members of the scientific community have important parts to play in forming research policy, carrying it out, and evaluating the results.

Second, academic teachers must include the concept of health for all in undergraduate, graduate and postgraduate training and continuing education. They must train many kinds of professionals to transform ideas and knowledge into action based on sound scientific evidence, if the targets are to be reached.

Third, the scientific community must give scientifically based, practical advice to the politicians and administrators responsible for decisions affecting people's health and welfare.

3

Promoting policies on research for health for all

To achieve their objectives, regional and country policies on research for health for all must win the support of the people who will make and implement them. Just as Member States must be persuaded to build their own policies, certain groups within each country need to be convinced of the worth of a country policy if they are to create and implement it. These groups include: the scientific community, agencies giving funds to research, and the authorities in charge of science, research and health.

Creating a country policy and making it work will require changes in the thought and work of all the different groups involved. Such a disruption of the way things are will naturally arouse opposition, particularly from the groups most closely concerned. A promotion strategy is needed to overcome the obstacles that will arise and win support for country policies by demonstrating their value and the advantages accompanying the changes.

Goal-directed research is new to many research workers. Some may believe that a policy based on such research attacks the principle of scientific and academic freedom. Research workers also have a different time frame from policy-makers and administrators, who are interested in applying rather than getting research results.

Obstacles

In addition, while fully recognizing the great contributions and potential of basic research, a policy on research for health for all will also emphasize applied research, health services research, and reseach using the methods and concepts of the social sciences. Part of the research community looks somewhat askance at such research. It can often be performed only in the country concerned and does not offer the research worker the chance to gain international recognition. In addition, reports on such research may not be able to cross the editorial threshold of the most prestigious scientific journals.

Policies on research for health for all also stress the use of existing knowledge. Although research workers are in the best position to point out the available knowledge on which any planned action could be based, neither they nor decision-makers may welcome such a public service. All too often, decision-makers request that more research be done, not to obtain more information but to delay action, especially in politically sensitive areas. Researchers who rob them of this excuse receive little intellectual satisfaction and less professional recognition.

Further, science and research are under the authority of their own ministry or that of education in most countries. Since the results of research for health for all are expected primarily to benefit the work of health ministries, people in other ministries will not be eager to devote their time to it. In addition, there will be the complex problem of coordinating the action needed from the other partners in the work: universities, foundations, industry and independent research institutions.

Finally, an important task of research for health for all is to find out why systems or programmes succeed or fail. As Socrates found, criticism of the *status quo* can be dangerous. Once launched, a health care programme, for example, will be very difficult to change, no matter the results of evaluative research. Too many vested interests, as well as much personal and professional prestige, are involved. On the other hand, too much is sometimes expected from a new type of research. People may expect that health systems or operational research, for instance, will cure all the ills of a health

42

care system. Research that fails to meet such expectations may be undeservedly discarded in the disappointment of the moment.

These obstacles and others like them can be overcome. Some, like the problems of organization, will be removed in the process of implementing the policy. Breaking down the others, however, will require that researchers, administrators, decision-makers and others wholeheartedly support the policy, deciding that its advantages for society and for themselves far outweigh the disadvantages.

The first step in winning support for a policy on research for health for all is to show that the policy is needed. This will be much easier in countries that have already made their own strategies for health for all and endorsed the regional targets. In these countries a policy on research for health for all is the logical next step. Other countries, however, must first be convinced of the need for health for all before they can be wooed to support such corollaries as a research policy. Ministries of health, education and science must cooperate in promoting the policies. WHO collaborating centres and non-governmental organizations can also give useful aid. **A promotion strategy**

After proving the need for a research policy, a promotion strategy must show that the regional policy or a particular country policy can fill that need. The strengths of a well constructed policy thus become proofs of its usefulness and powerful tools in promotion. It will naturally be much easier to promote a policy that is:

- practical, scientifically sound and easy to understand;

- an essential part of the country's policies on health for all and on general health research;

- developed and implemented by people from a wide range of disciplines, particularly researchers; and

- made more flexible and useful by its evaluation component.

Member States and WHO can do much, separately and together, to promote policies on research for health for all. Most of the activities described as promotional, however, actually serve two *Marketing research policies*

43

purposes. They do more than promote research policies: they help to build and implement them.

For example, all of the six promotional activities suggested for Member States will be just as essential to creating and carrying out a research policy. Member States should: make statements supporting research for health for all, involve and consult researchers in the development of the policy, help the generators and users of research findings to communicate, involve other bodies at the appropriate level in carrying out the policy, identify the prerequisites for high-priority research, and spread the news of the policy to all the people concerned.

Several of the activities intended for WHO also serve this double purpose. These include work to stimulate and assist countries to develop their own policies and research for health for all (such as this book), to coordinate international cooperative ventures, and to establish a network of European universities to work for health for all.

Further, WHO can promote both research policies, and the communication needed to make them work, in a number of ways. First, the Organization should consider establishing a clearinghouse for research policies and studies for health for all, and publishing a newsletter on the topic. In addition, the network of WHO collaborating centres should be used to spread information about different country policies, to conduct the recommended research and to share the results. WHO should also hold meetings for representatives of other intergovernmental agencies conducting health-related research, nongovernmental scientific organizations, scientific and professional journals, and science and research administrations in countries (health and social research councils). WHO could give further help by standardizing research terminology, indicators and methods, and by aligning its own research activities with country research for health for all. In addition, WHO should collaborate with other international agencies to promote and implement research for health for all.

Finally, Member States and WHO should cooperate to make research policies work. Government authorities, WHO and the members of the European Advisory Committee on Health Research should spread and promote the ideas behind the health for all movement through all available channels, including the mass media. In addition, Member States and WHO should:

— convene liaison meetings to bring together the producers and potential users of the results of research for health for all;

— forestall potential obstacles to the acceptance of regional and country policies on research for health for all; and

— encourage the developers of research policies to write and submit articles about them to scientific and professional journals.

Promoting policies on research for health for all is yet another task in which cooperation is the key.

Regional and country strategies for research for health for all must measure their success by the changes they bring about in countries. They will have achieved their goals if Member States progress towards the following ideal state of affairs.

Signs of success

● All Member States develop their own strategies and policies for research for health for all, in line with their own and regional health for all policies.

● The research community widens the scope of its work to include areas of high priority in achieving health for all.

● Research councils and private foundations include the funding of such research in their policies.

● Personnel working in high-priority areas have adequate opportunities for research training.

● Talented young researchers can be assured of a career when they undertake research for health for all.

45

- Scientific journals are receptive to research for health for all.

- Researchers spell out the implications of their findings for health policy.

- Decision-makers, administrators and planners actively seek scientific evidence as a basis for their decisions, plans and actions.